QUANTUM HEALING WITH NUTRITION

HELEN BARNSHAW

Disclaimer

This book is not intended as a substitute for a 1-1 nutritional therapy program. The reader should regularly consult a therapist in matters relating to his/her health and particularly with respect to any symptoms that may require diagnosis or medical attention.

Copyright © Helen Barnshaw

All rights reserved. No part of this book may be reproduced or used in any manner without the prior written permission of the copyright owner, except for the use of brief quotations in a book review.

Hardcover: 978-1-64746-688-6
Paperback: 978-1-64746-687-9
Ebook: 978-1-64746-689-3

Library of Congress Number: 2021901344

First paperback edition March 2021.

Edited by the AAE Guild
Cover art by JetLaunch
Layout by JetLaunch

Printed by KDP in the USA.

https://helenbarnshaw.podia.com

TABLE OF CONTENTS

Introduction 1

NUTRITIONAL SCIENCE 5

Chapter 1   Your Body Already Knows
             How to Heal Itself. 7
Chapter 2   The Importance of Balance 9
Chapter 3   Why Naturopathy? 12
Chapter 4   Epigenetics and Influencing Your Genes
             for Better Health 15
Chapter 5   How a Personalized Program Helps You to
             Reach Your Fullest Potential in Healing
             and Happiness. 18
Chapter 6   Natural Remedies 21
Chapter 7   The Gut/Mind Connection. 25
Chapter 8   What Are Some of the Early Warning Signs
             of Chronic Stress and Disease? 28
Chapter 9   Gluten and Wheat Testing for the Earliest
             Prevention of Autoimmune Disease. 30
Chapter 10   Cleansing and Probiotics in the Story of
             Restoring the Microbiome. 34
Chapter 11   Intro to Superpower Wholefoods. 36
Chapter 12   Healthier Treat Foods 40

Chapter 13   Powerful Tips for Commencing the Reversal
              of Chronic Disease Symptoms Right Now... 42
Chapter 14   Testimonials 44

SPIRITUAL DEVELOPMENT GUIDANCE.......47

Chapter 15   Intention and Visualization for
              Setting Off on the Right Path 49
Chapter 16   Meditation to Support Lasting Influence
              on Your Mind 52
Chapter 17   Self-Acceptance and Self-Compassion:
              Making the Healing Process Easier 56

HABIT-BUILDING TOOLS FOR HEALING 59

Chapter 18   How Physical Tools Make it Easier
              to Build Positive Habits................. 61

About the Author................................67

APPENDICES 71

Bibliography 73
Additional Tools and Resources 75
Online Program.................................77
Endorsements 79

INTRODUCTION

A quantum healing guide to address stress, reverse illness, prevent disease, and discover your deepest happiness and potential, using whole foods.

This guide brings together the best spiritual, scientific, and habit-building techniques, to heal anyone wanting to reach full potential in health and happiness, using wholefoods and natural medicine.

We look at how Asian and Western knowledge have evolved and combined to what we understand as nutritional therapy, naturopathic nutrition and functional medicine practices today.

The information in this book is designed to provide you with the most effective methods for healing from chronic disease and preventing it altogether. They have been tried and tested and are designed to meet you wherever you are with your own personal healing journey at this time. Whether you're thinking of getting started with a nutritional therapist or are already on a healing journey, included are all of the aspects which have propelled myself and my clients to fuller healing. These are broken down into three sections:

Nutritional Science—The scientific knowledge part of healing with nutrition.

Spiritual Development Guidance—The emotional growth tools and the foundation to deeper healing, which helps us to let go of the negative habits that have kept us in a bad place. This allows us to develop sustainable health and happiness long-term.

Habit-Building Tools for Healing—Specific strategies that will bring your new learning into the physical realm for healing now, helping you leap into achieving the health and happiness you are worthy of sooner.

HOW IS THIS BOOK GOING TO HELP ME ON MY HEALING JOURNEY USING FUNCTIONAL FOODS?

This book will teach you how to build self-compassion and acceptance, how to allow yourself to accept support from multiple sources, how this supports faster healing, and how this brings us more power over our happiness and well-being long into the future. It is designed to be a helping hand to those embarking on a healing journey through becoming a nutritional therapist or as a client of a nutritional therapy program. It is designed to support you in building the mindset and habits of a healing warrior—whether you're healing yourself or want to become a healer for others. I talk about mindset, meditation, help setting intention, support in achieving balance, we talk about tools to support you to achieve building positive habits faster, the benefits of natural healing and embarking on a nutritional therapy program, also known as naturopathic nutrition, whole foods healing, and functional foods healing. Most importantly this book will allow you to fully enjoy the process of healing with whole foods. It offers a full complement to any nutritional therapy program, supporting you in building a strong mindset and habits, which will facilitate your success in achieving faster symptom relief and enabling fuller healing on a cellular level.

On a naturopathic nutrition journey, you experience lasting progressive healing. You are joining the many who have

INTRODUCTION

embarked on an evolved way of thinking and being. You are becoming part of the future. You are stepping away from the traditional methods you once relied on, which once kept you in a small and stagnant place mentally, physically, and emotionally.

As I continue to share my learning with you and supporting you with your healing, I continue to see higher and more sustained happiness as you and others begin to take back control of your lives through fast and healthy symptom relief, reversing illness, preventing disease, losing weight healthily and easily, and restoring mobility and independence. You are worthy of experiencing complete happiness and health, fulfilling your highest potential and enjoying your life to the fullest.

NUTRITIONAL SCIENCE

1
YOUR BODY ALREADY KNOWS HOW TO HEAL ITSELF

Your body has an amazing ability to protect you from harmful microbes and substances like viruses, bacteria, fungi, and parasites. When you can learn to work with it, you can help to optimize its healing power.

Your body is already equipped with the natural ability to protect you through powerful functions, which help to keep harmful substances out of the body. You know these exist through the specific immune system and non-specific immune system. Our non-specific immune defence system comes in the form of our skin. As the largest organ in the human body, it acts as a barrier from harmful substances entering the body. Phagocytes are organisms, which engulf and destroy any invading organisms. They are found in many of our organs such as the liver, lungs, and intestinal tract. Natural killer cells recognize cells that have been invaded by viruses. They bind to these cells and destroy them. Your specific immune system is your body's ability to produce antibodies throughout the process of recognizing and destroying harmful cells. The antibody does the job of recognizing the harmful cell and phagocytes and then destroy that part of the cell. Antibodies are made by white blood cells called B lymphocytes within the immune system. These come in thousands of varieties of strains, specifically for recognizing different antigen markers.

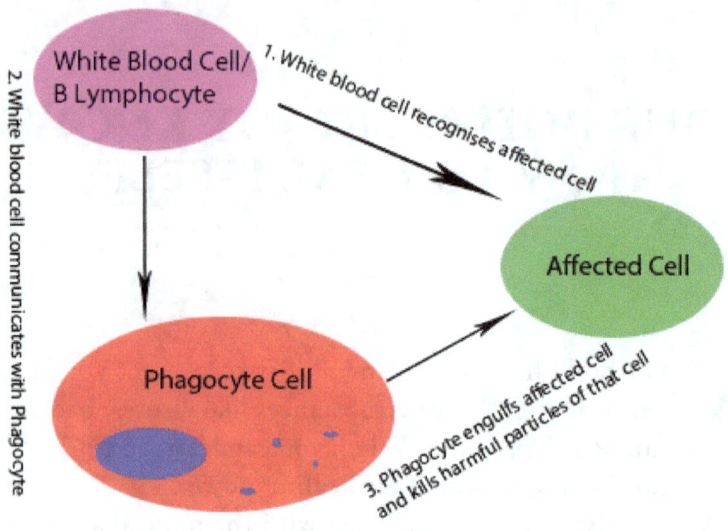

Fig 1.1, Phagocytosis diagram. Copywrite Helen Barnshaw

Learning to understand and work with your body is easier than you think. Throughout this book I will help you to learn and optimize your health to achieve the highest mental, physical, emotional, and social well-being possible. You have nothing to lose here!

2
THE IMPORTANCE OF BALANCE

Balance in all things is crucial. When it comes to your body, it already has natural intelligence within its core cells to sustain this balance; it is your lifestyle and environment that are the controlling factors between health and disease. When you have the right knowledge and will to succeed, you truly hold the power to your own health and happiness.

Chinese naturopathy has always fascinated me, and I believe they discovered the answers to balanced and healthier living centuries before western society. While studying to earn my Western Naturopathic Nutrition diploma, I was often able to recognize elements of Asian nutrition beliefs and tips popping up throughout the studies.

Asian naturopathy, specifically Chinese naturopathy, invented the use of yin and yang as a way to better understand and equate balance in health and living. They created a term for the energy of all things, called qi (pronounced *chee*) which refers to the vitality and energy within a person. Qi holds the essence of yang, which is responsible for warming elements of food, air, and organs in the body, representing movement. Yin is the opposite of yang and is responsible for all cold aspects representing stagnancy and blockage. It focuses on cold, interior, and deficiency. Yang conversely revolves around heat, exterior, and excess. An example of this relationship in food is the use of raw food, which is considered to have cooling effects on the body. Cooked food eaten cold also has a cooling effect. Hot foods have a warming and moving effect on the body.

Seeing warming and cooling elements as yin and yang helps you to better gauge the effects of certain foods on the human body. Too much of any one element will cause an unbalanced stasis. Therefore, yin and yang is, and has been for some centuries, a helpful gauge in keeping a balance in health and lifestyle.

Aelius Galenus, also known as Galen, was a Greek physician, writer, and philosopher during the period circa 130 AD to circa 210 AD. He created the understanding of the four humours.

Humour theory (meaning juice or sap), is the concept which states all four of the humours are to be kept in balance. These humours are blood, black bile, yellow bile, and phlegm, and Galen developed theories for how various foods affect the humours differently. If someone was suffering from phlegmatic symptoms, warm, dry foods would help to rebalance the body. When one or more of these humours comes out of balance, disease prevails. Galen created purging, bloodletting, cupping, and emetics, as curative measures to help keep humours in balance.

Current science and complementary medicine have now advanced so far as to recognize the importance of maintaining a balance in everything. You can better understand now how many aspects are responsible for your health. The study of epigenetics dives into the effects of the environment, food, and upbringing on cellular changes within your body, focusing on family history, genetics, birth environment, upbringing, lifestyle, diet, mental health, learned habits, and exercise. We will talk more about this in Chapter 4: Epigenetics and Influencing Your Genes for Better Health.

Homoeostasis is the state of the body's systems constantly rebalancing itself from internal and external factors. As defined by Walter Cannon in the late 1800s, "Constancy in an open system, such as our bodies represent, requires mechanisms acting to maintain this constancy." (Walter Cannon in Biochemical Imbalances in Disease, p30). Homeostasis helps you to understand how the body is made up of many cooperating systems working together to keep the body regulated among states of constant change. When the amount of work your body has to do to keep this healthy balance is overloaded, illness or disease can set in. In functional medicine, this stage is called allostasis, a condition proposed by Peter Sterling and Joseph Eyer in 1988.

With so much historical knowledge and current scientific research, you have all the evidence and support you need to make the right decisions in living a more balanced lifestyle. Food, exercise, and mental health are some of the most influential factors within your control. You have the power to keep these elements in balance, ensuring a healthy and happy life.

3
WHY NATUROPATHY?

When you have tried everything in front of you to heal and nothing has helped, when you want a better solution and feel there has to be something more sustainable, you are right—there is something beyond the traditional methods in current medicine. Those of you who have been brave enough to step beyond yourselves have discovered more evolved and faster ways to heal—and it requires an acceptance of where you are now and believing that there is a better way to heal beyond what you know.

Traditional medicine has come a long way since the beginning. It has given us a way to tackle disease, reduce pain, restore needed cells, and more. It has evolved as you have and offers a powerful way to help stop illness in its tracks if you use it right. Medicine was only ever meant to be used as a temporary support to help reduce the symptoms and not to tackle the cause. The thought processes encompassing traditional medicine, which you've been brought up with, are not for the purpose of tackling the cause of disease and sustaining health for the longer term.

There are a handful of early doctors and physicians who began to discover better ways to treat patients that went beyond

NUTRITIONAL SCIENCE

traditional medicine. They were the founders and early influencers of naturopathic medicine.

Hippocrates, born circa 460 BC, separated illness from religion, establishing that illness is the product of living habits, diet, and environment. He asserted that the human body has the power to rebalance itself when treated within the right environment. Dr. Pierre Charles Alexandre Louis (1787–1872) introduced the concept that the knowledge and history of a disease could be found using clinical trials. His work, which represents the earliest accounts of clinical trials, involved taking detailed case histories to build a more complete picture. He believed that the physician's role was to do everything possible to help people to recover naturally from disease. In 1854 Florence Nightingale (1820–1920), discovered that the unsanitary conditions of the Crimean war hospital barracks contributed to ten times more deaths than the war itself. She eventually trained nurses and hospitals to improve their cleanliness, which brought better sanitation, better sewer and enhanced ventilation. She also understood that diet and activity were important to help the human body in its job of healing, and she was able to largely reduce the mortality rate during that time. She knew that the body and mind work together to heal and that improving lifestyle habits and cleanliness in the environment supported the body's natural ability to do its job of healing.

Jeremy Narby is an anthropologist who is interested in a kind of intelligence other than the one you see and experience in your mind. In his book, *Intelligence in Nature*, Narby does a great job of proving that your cells contain another form of intelligence and that this is the reason you are here today. It is the intuition you often try to ignore and is the ever-evolving nature that continues regardless of the knowledge typically viewed as intelligence. Narby goes on to explain how slime moulds solve mazes, bees handle abstract concepts, and plants gauge the world around them. These are all living organisms that do not have a human brain, yet they have a knowing—a cellular intelligence that holds knowledge and supports them in learning and discovering as they live. Narby also talks about how Macaws along the Urubamba River in South America all gather once a day to eat clay. He discovered that the clay holds vital nutrients that help them to detoxify harmful substances found in the seeds which they eat; by binding to these substances, it helps to speed up elimination from the birds' body. Their cells have an intuition, a knowing of what it requires to keep surviving.

What I am trying to demonstrate here is there is a higher knowledge and intelligence within your body. Your cells hold an empirical knowledge that can help you to survive. It's all knowing and separate from your mind's intelligence. To access this higher knowledge, you must let go of the restrictive expectations of using only your mind's intelligence to heal. The trick is to achieve a balance between what your body is guiding you to do and how your mind can support you in achieving this.

In the next chapter, I will discuss how current nutrition science recognizes the intelligence in your cells and how environmental factors influence them to express themselves in different ways—epigenetics.

4
EPIGENETICS AND INFLUENCING YOUR GENES FOR BETTER HEALTH

Epigenetics explains how important every aspect of your life is to your cells. Lifestyles, environments, food, thoughts, feelings, and people all influence the current state of your cells to express themselves in various ways. With this knowledge, you are able to make changes to aspects of your life, which will move your cells' behaviour towards positive changes to your health and how you permanently feel.

You are born into this world with a set of genes that act as instructions descended from early man and are slowly modified through generations. You are the most evolved form of the human genome. With every single environmental, emotional, and physical challenge, your cells are forced to develop strategies to help you survive. If these strategies are successful for survival in long-term environments, your genes are forced to favour these responses for longer-term survival, which over a long period of time eventually become genetic changes. As a result, your environment influences your cells and ultimately leads to evolution.

Epigenetics looks at how external factors affect the way in which a gene expresses itself in favourable and unfavourable circumstances, without changing the genetic code itself. It works through chemical tags added to chromosomes, which switch genes on and off. There are various mice studies demonstrating this by using tightly controlled laboratory conditions to reveal how epigenetics work with phenotypes and methyl tags. The best study, in my opinion, is one in which Kerry Ressler—a neurobiologist and psychiatrist in Atlanta, Georgia and his colleague Brian Dias—became interested in epigenetic inheritance in impoverished and poverty-stricken people after working with some in cities who took to drug addiction and showed signs of neurological illness. They found these behaviours were also learned from their parents or passed along to their children.

Ressler and Dias decided to study epigenetic inheritance in laboratory mice, training them to fear the smell of almonds and cherries (acetophenone). They did this by using electric shocks on the mice while wafting acetophenone around them. Eventually the mice learned to associate the smell with something terrible. Their reaction was eventually passed onto their pups. The scientists were able to demonstrate that even though the pups had never encountered acetophenone, they still exhibited increased sensitivity when introduced to the smell, in comparison to other mice who had been trained using another smell or who had no conditioning at all. The studies also showed these reactions could also be passed down from the grandmother's generation.

Knowing what your body needs and doesn't need gives you the power to be able to influence your own gene expression for better health. You have a unique gene sequence, which translates into different metabolisms, growth rate, energy, and enzyme production. Take two completely different people and give them the exact same lifestyles and their bodies will react differently as they're made up of different genes requiring different things to survive. On the other end of the spectrum, take a pair of twins who are made up of very similar genes, but this time give them completely different lifestyles, and you'll see their bodies begin to look different almost immediately.

5

HOW A PERSONALIZED PROGRAM HELPS YOU TO REACH YOUR FULLEST POTENTIAL IN HEALING AND HAPPINESS

Nutritional therapy outlines the causes and effects of your lifestyle and habits on your health. It provides a framework and consultative support to get you on the right track to better health and happiness, which is sustainable long into your future. Food is one of the most influential factors on your body. If you are looking to improve your health in some way, doing it through nutrition is an effective and powerful way to begin influencing your body's health.

Nutritional therapy takes your current nutrition habits and lifestyle, and—combined with reading internal and external bodily symptoms—understands why your body has been brought out of balance and what is required to restore balance. It also provides you with the framework and support to sustain and build better health for continued, more developed happiness for your future. There are no limits to the level of health and happiness you can achieve. All it takes is an understanding that this exists and an acceptance of the support available and you can achieve anything. As we discussed in previous chapters, you first need to believe there are other more evolved ways to help you heal more effectively that exist outside of the traditional healthcare framework.

Do you have ambition for more fulfilled happiness now and in the future? Do you wish to fulfil your dreams? Take a look on Instagram and other social media platforms all around you, and you will see this is even more achievable for you now than, say, 10 years ago, as you are provided with the framework and tools to recognize and achieve your highest potential as a more evolved human being. There are so many accessible resources out there for you now. When you are able to focus on keeping your health and happiness in check, you are able to more easily achieve other things you put your mind to. Your health is a vital key to achieving that potential. Without it you are not able to help others. Think of those now-familiar safety instructions that airplane passengers hear prior to taking off— secure your own oxygen mask first and then assist others. Without taking that step, you are at risk of collapsing, even dying, which would render you completely useless to those around you.

A nutritional therapy program first takes into account your family and personal health history. This gives a more specific and focused diagnosis on your current health. It then takes into consideration your current health habits from the food you eat, your sleeping habits, exercise rates, and stress levels as well as any current internal and external symptoms. These symptoms are read to understand what nutrients you are deficient in then, combined with the knowledge of your family history and current personal habits, we are able to understand exactly how these deficiencies have come about. A diet strategy methodology can then be drawn up, demonstrating how to easily access and imbibe the relevant nutrients your body requires and how to speed up and strengthen the absorption of these nutrients for the most efficient healing possible.

Follow the web link at the end of this book, for more tools and resources.

6
NATURAL REMEDIES

There are limitless options for reducing symptoms of illness when you allow yourself to look beyond the confines of what you already know. Natural herbs and tinctures have been used to heal human symptoms for centuries. Although medication can be an effective way to initially slow down chronic pain, because of its man-made structure it is not designed to address the cause of the illness or help your body heal beyond reducing symptoms.

Many types of herbs and spices can be used to reduce all types of symptoms, from muscle pain, to headaches, to period pain. I have liked using them in the form of a hot tea tonic, which allows the body to digest them faster and allows the nutrients to be more effectively absorbed into the bloodstream for rapid relief. Tinctures are an effective way to reduce symptoms, for long-term health our aim is to reduce the occurrence of the illness in the first place. This is achieved through a good balance of healthy eating, rest, and exercise. When you are healthier, you are able to achieve higher levels of life satisfaction and happiness because you're able to physically and mentally do what you want to do.

Medication is a man-made treatment for pain, disease, and diagnosis. It is made from various cellular strains that have had their molecular structure manipulated for the purpose of human consumption. Traditional medicine was designed to relieve pain, but no emphasis was made to help patients heal the causes of their pain in order to fully heal. Many disease patients are led to believe that the medication is then their only source of staying alive, and they become completely reliant on the treatment. The key is to understand we all have control over our own health and happiness and can all heal and become self-reliant in doing so. Treatment or medication from the traditional healthcare framework can then be used as an emergency, temporary measure if required.

Because medication is man-made, the human body is often unable to completely absorb the cells. This can build up in your liver and kidneys as excess waste, which puts pressure on your organs to fully perform as waste removal experts. If your body is unable to successfully excrete any excess waste and toxins, these will build up in your blood and fat cells then put pressure on your heart. As you can see, this is completely the wrong way to go about healing yourself for the longer term. It is more easily demonstrated through the popular use of protein supplements for bodybuilding. They help the body to build more muscle but as a result they leave excess protein build up in the liver because the human body can only absorb a small amount of protein at any one time. Because this excess protein hasn't been able to metabolise, it causes a build-up of nitrogenous waste in the blood stream, which damages the kidneys and the heart and creates a higher risk of cancer. This is only a supplemental example, so you can imagine the damage from excess medication. It is known that long-term use of pain relief medication can directly damage and slow down the kidneys and the heart; and without your kidneys, your body is unable to detox.

For patients on heavy medication, you can get the support of a nutritional therapist together with your doctor, to learn how to safely reduce your medications, as you are on the quest for real healing. The benefits of replacing some medications with natural remedies is threefold: 1) you still get the symptom and pain relief required but with no toxic build up; 2) it is more accepted in the human body; and 3) when used as part of a nutrition therapy program tailored specifically to your body's needs, it can be an extremely effective and fast way to heal on a cellular level.

You might already have some effective herbs in your kitchen cupboard, which will reduce your pain just as effectively as medication. There are numerous books and blogs out there that can teach you more about natural remedies alone. You can find a plethora of these on Amazon when you search for natural home remedies. Here are a few helpful nuggets to get you started:

- Chamomile: Calms your digestive system and mind when imbibed orally. When used externally, it can soothe skin irritation and rashes.
- Nettle: Cleanses your digestive tract, reduces blood sugar, lowers cholesterol, and supports heart health. It is also said to reduce prostate inflammation.
- Dandelion Leaf: One of my faves! I have used it on myself and my clients have also used it to help reduce symptoms of inflammation and pain; it is especially useful for cleansing the blood to help reduce rheumatic pain. I have also used it to reduce period pain.
- Peppermint: Good for digestion, freshens breath, helps fight infection, relieves clogged sinuses and improves energy.
- Raspberry Leaf: Has been used for decades as a womb toner to improve birthing conditions. I have used it

in the past to successfully reduce symptoms of period pain.
- Green Tea: A powerful antioxidant. The polyphenols in green tea help fight oxidative stress in the body.
- Ginger: Is high in magnesium, sodium, vitamin C and vitamin B6. It is so versatile and can be used in many types of drinks, and desserts. It is a powerful antioxidant helping to strengthen the immune system, reduce inflammation, fight infection, reduce blood sugar, and lower cholesterol. I always have ginger in my cupboard as it can be used in many ways.
- Lemon: This is a fruit and not an herb, but it is a versatile antioxidant, you can add to many drinks and in cooking. I always add a touch of lemon to my vodka and tonic, not just for taste but also to add a cleansing element to my drink. It is also very effective in making make your own mixes, using tea bags or loose leaves—whatever works best for you as a fast remedy.

7
THE GUT/MIND CONNECTION

The vagus nerve is one of the largest nerves in your body. It runs from your brainstem to other parts of your body, with the importance of receiving and monitoring information about various functions throughout your whole body. It does such a great job connecting your gut and mind together, when one is out of balance it affects the other. Bacteria and viruses in the gut affect the chemical messages passing between the two. Just as with the mind, if emotional or physical disturbance is present, it can affect the function of your gut. You may have noticed when you're in a stressful situation at work or home—due to the fight or flight response—the body will shut down particular functions in order to support the body through these stressful situations. One of the functions it shuts down is digestive ability. As you begin to learn and understand the relationship between the two, you will have the power to support more efficient healing, through nurturing both.

Nurture the mind with:

- Good quality sleep for at least eight hours a night by developing a regular routine your body will get used to.
- Clean eating and feel-good nutrients that support the brain's function; B vitamins, particularly B12, support the brain's growth and development. Find these in fish, nuts, and seeds.
- Green tea and berries, which contain phytochemicals and vitamin C to support cleansing and bring clarity and focus.
- Adaptogens like ashwagandha, ginseng, and turmeric that support the body by reducing the symptoms of stress. Natural stimulants like caffeine and ginseng boost brain function by blocking adenosine, a neurotransmitter responsible for making you sleepy—these should be imbibed in small amounts.
- B vitamins and small amounts of natural stimulants that promote the feel-good chemicals serotonin, norepinephrine, and dopamine. These chemicals are made in the gut.

Nurture the gut with:

- Probiotics to support its natural function. These are live bacteria and yeasts supporting the digestive function. The main bacteria are firmicutes, bacteroidetes, actinobacteria, and proteobacteria. You also can boost the strains of lactobacillus and bifidobacterium through probiotic capsules. Freeze-dried powder form is proven to be more effective, as it activates as soon as it hits the gut juices.
- A light detox to boost your body's ability to fight toxins and begin healing faster. Always consult a nutritional

practitioner or doctor before commencing a cleanse, so you can understand the best one for your body type and be aware of any risks for patients on high amounts of medication. Dandelion leaf tea is an example of an herb that deeply cleanses the digestive system and liver, thus cleansing the blood and reducing prostaglandins, which are the direct result of the pain response.
- Foods like yogurt, bananas, kefir, and fermented foods—known as prebiotics, which support good bacteria in the digestive system—that contain compounds to induce the growth of beneficial bacteria and fungi.

As Jeremy Narby explains on his quest for understanding the natural intelligence of the human body, "the brain is not limited to the skull. My gut alone contains about one hundred million neutrons capable of learning, remembering, and responding to emotions, just like the larger brain in my head." There are tissue networks of neutrons lining the oesophagus, stomach, small intestine, and colon, connecting the gut and the head.

8
WHAT ARE SOME OF THE EARLY WARNING SIGNS OF CHRONIC STRESS AND DISEASE?

This book is designed to meet you wherever you are with your healing journey, whether you want to reverse symptoms or prevent them. Preventing disease is obviously the most powerful way to avoid disease early on. You can learn, however, to recognize and stop any symptoms in their tracks before they lead to disease.

Poor habits, if repeated with consistency over long periods, will eventually lead to disease. Your body needs you to take care of it. The challenge you have is realizing, learning, and maintaining a healthy balance in life so you can enjoy it to its fullest and ensure it for years to come. Investing in your health has never been easier now with technology making resources more accessible.

What are some of the signs of stress?

- Poor sleep
- Overeating
- Over imbibing toxins like alcohol, drugs, and smoking
- Over working
- Depression
- Anxiety

What are the symptoms?

- Fatigue and tiredness
- Feeling low and depressed
- Feeling under or over satiated (not feeling full after eating or always wanting to eat)
- Irritable Bowel Syndrome—stomach cramps, diarrhoea, constipation, which are worsened with stress, and particular foods (more about this in the next chapter).
- Headaches
- Muscle pains or aches

Download the instant Stress Test and get help reducing your symptoms, through my online courses at *helenbarnshaw.podia.com*

9
GLUTEN AND WHEAT TESTING FOR THE EARLIEST PREVENTION OF AUTOIMMUNE DISEASE

As you now know, the gut is the most important part of the story when it comes to health. It is responsible for breaking down food, filtering toxins, and assimilating nutrients into the bloodstream. If the lining of the stomach or intestines are swollen and damaged, it can't properly do its job of breaking down food, assimilating nutrients, and keeping toxins out of the bloodstream. When this happens, toxin levels begin to rise and compromise the immune system. Over time things worsen and become harder to reverse as the immune system breaks down and can no longer protect the body from further pathogen damage. This leads to immune diseases. Recognizing any digestive issues early on gives you the power to prevent disease.

Many digestive issues start with the common symptoms of Irritable Bowel Syndrome, or IBS. They are:

- Painful abdominal spasms and/or cramps
- Bloating
- Constipation
- Problems emptying your bowel
- Loose stools or diarrhoea
- Flatulence
- Mucus or slime in the stools
- Blood in your stools
- Unexplained weight loss
- Anxiety or depression
- Stress

As well as treating the symptoms, treating the causes will prevent any further toxin build up and will greatly reduce your chances of developing immune diseases in the future. All the knowledge in the world won't help you unless you are able to recognize the habits which led you to where you are. Your habits have been built through ancestry, upbringing, and environmental challenges, so it will take dedication and patience to see these changes through.

Reducing toxins like excess caffeine, alcohol, smoking, over-medication, carbonated drinks, refined sugar, and processed food is the best way to start the process of healing. The next step is to look at your physical habits like sleep, exercise, and stress. Stress has some of the most negative influences on the digestive system. It is well known the body is programmed to shut down during stressful situations, in order to prioritize the blood flowing to the brain and nervous system. It follows that stress is damaging for digestion and health.

The next step is to eradicate any foods that directly irritate your gut. Gluten and wheat are usually the culprits here. Doing a gluten test on yourself using non-wheat foods such as cold cuts, ketchup, mayonnaise, soy sauce, or gravy will tell you if you are gluten intolerant, which is called celiac disease.

If you have no reaction to this gluten, then it could be that you are wheat allergic only—in which case, you can do a test on yourself by eating a wheat-heavy meal and monitor any symptoms that occur. You can also get a urine test performed by your local general practitioner to confirm this is so. Wheat gluten is found in many grains and not just wheat flour. It is also found in barley, rye, semolina, spelt, and many other grains.

These gluten-free grains are also good options:

- Buckwheat
- Corn
- Flaxseed
- Gram flour
- Hemp
- Millet
- Polenta
- Quinoa
- Rice
- Sesame
- Soya
- Tapioca
- Teff

There are many more out there, but these are the most accessible gluten-free grains on the market at the moment.

It is also worth noting that other symptoms of intolerance include lactose intolerance (dairy), and FODMAPs (fermentable oligo-saccharides, di-saccharides, mono-saccharides and polyols), which in simple terms means slow fermenting sugars, affecting those with a build-up of bad bacteria in the gut and making it harder for them to digest carbohydrates. There are other intolerances out there. Lactose and FODMAP intolerances are not immune responses but caused by a lack of something, which causes a sensitivity response. If left without proper recognition or treatment they can eventually become more serious and may cause an immune response and eventual illness, as the digestive system becomes damaged and unable to assimilate nutrients and appropriately block toxins to protect the body. There are some simple tests you can do on yourself here or you can get functional tests performed by your doctor so you can be sure and start to get clearer on your next steps for healing. I can also support you here too, but as IBS is a more serious immune response that can quickly spiral out of control and cause other immune diseases fast, I have chosen to prioritize writing about this to immediately help those most in distress and at risk. If you'd like to get in touch for a one-on-one nutritional therapy program to support any of the conditions I have discussed, you can find more details on my website. The link will be provided at the end of this book.

For more severe symptoms of pain and stress, it is advised to seek the support of a nutritional therapy program, so you have artillery of healing tools specific to your requirements. This will bring you the most optimal healing, as you allow your body to heal on a deeper cellular level. Get access to a Wheat & Gluten Intolerance Testing sheet, and more on my website at *helenbarnshaw.podia.com*

10
CLEANSING AND PROBIOTICS IN THE STORY OF RESTORING THE MICROBIOME

You understand now that your body already knows how to heal itself. When you reduce your bad habits and toxins going into your body, you immediately help your body to begin the healing process. In Chapter 2, we discussed homeostasis and how your body is always striving to keep you in a balanced state. When your body becomes overloaded with toxins from external factors and food, it enters into a state of allostasis where it is fighting to bring back the balance.

When you are able to recognize any symptoms of stress and illness, you can immediately reduce toxin intake and bad habits, which have created the imbalance, and begin the healing process. See Chapter 13 for more detail on recognizing symptoms and tips for preventing illness and beginning the reversal of disease.

Cleansing is an important step in the story to helping your body to heal and is something your body already knows how to do. Your body already performs a fasting process whilst you sleep; this occurs during the period between dinner and breakfast the next day. When you sleep, your body is in rest phase with reduced heart rate and use of organs and muscles. This is when it works to cleanse toxins and repair any cell damage. You can support this process for your body by inducing more cleansing through fasting activities like juice, water, or pulse cleansing depending on your body type and needs.

How can I help my body to cleanse?

- Stop toxin intake and reduce consumption of bad foods.
- Begin taking a probiotic capsule every morning. This builds on our gut's natural ability to break down foods and cleanse. The capsules should include various strains such as lactobacillus and bifidobacterium cultures.
- Get more sleep to allow more opportunity for natural cleansing and cell rebuilding.
- Plan a regular weekly or monthly cleanse, depending on the severity of your condition.
- Implement tonics with healing herbs and spices, which reduce symptoms of pain.
- Eat foods with the specific nutrients your body needs to excel the cellular healing process.

I have performed many fasts on myself and helped clients to implement fasts specifically tailored to their needs. Not only does it immediately begin the healing process, but you begin to feel the benefits straight away. Cleansing reduces toxins, also reducing the inflammatory responses, which cause pain (prostaglandin production). You will begin to feel reduced pain and feel more alert as brain fog clears; and you feel happy and more energetic as your body can now begin to assimilate good nutrients faster. For help with fasting safely, healing & strengthening your immune system, and reducing stress & anxiety, download my supporting tools and get access to my courses, all found on my website at *helenbarnshaw.podia.com*

11
INTRO TO SUPERPOWER WHOLEFOODS

All foods are a combination of different particles, naturally formed. Any combination is possible. Some foods, especially those that are man-made, might contain little to no nutritional substance, meaning it is hard for your body to convert and make good use of them. If your body is unable to find good use for the particles, it will class them as waste material, which deposits itself as a toxin in your body. Other foods have a better balance of nutrients, while some contain a favourable mixture of detoxifying qualities and nutritious value. These foods are therefore known for their amazing ability to help your body to heal faster.

Yellow fruit and vegetables contain carotenoids and beta-carotene, which convert to Vitamin A, for eye, skin, and immune system health.

Dark fruits and vegetables (like berries, peppers, red onions) contain polyphenols (a kind of phytonutrient), which are packed with antioxidants and nutrients supporting digestion, weight management, reduces diabetes, and reduces cardiovascular disease. Polyphenols are also found in green and white tea.

Green leafy vegetables contain large amounts of chlorophyll, which is a form of antioxidant. Chlorophyll in green foods help to detoxify the blood, aid wound healing, gut health, energy, support the immune system, and help to prevent cancer.

Microalgae are known for their high amount of chlorophyll and healing nutrients, specifically protein and DNA lipids that heal the very core of our nervous system and brain. Microalgae also contains other B vitamins, magnesium, calcium, iron, potassium, and vitamin E. These are all important for supporting muscles, energy, and growth of new cells. Microalgae is so powerful it has been used by the Amazonians to heal the sick for centuries. Now Western society can find various strains of microalgae in a powder form to suit individual needs in shops or online. I get mine from Amazon, funnily enough.

Microalgae has actually played a powerful role in my life and in the story of some of my clients' healing; it is packed with antioxidants and nutrients, which helps to speed up the healing process in our bodies. There are, however, many different strains which contain different make ups of micronutrients and antioxidants, and getting the right one for your body type is very important to support a healthy cleanse and faster repair without becoming undernourished. Chlorella, for example, contains protein and healthy lipids to build muscle tissue and support the nervous system. This is better for smaller framed bodies. Spirulina and wild blue-green algae contain slightly smaller amounts of these nutrients but are still powerful enough as a healing substance.

There is also wheatgrass. You can get this in powder, juice, and capsule form. Wheatgrass has many of the nutrients that microalgae contains and has larger amounts of antioxidants and cleansing cells, which are effective for larger frames requiring more of a detox. I have used this for more than six years, and although it's not to be used every day, it supports me to start off a deep cleanse when I feel my body needs it. I always use it once a month, at least one week before my period starts, as it boosts my body with the nutrients that it uses up the most throughout the menstrual cycle; these are magnesium, B vitamins, vitamin E, iron and zinc. Wheatgrass contains potassium, dietary fibre, vitamin A, vitamin C, vitamin E (alpha tocopherol), vitamin K, thiamine, riboflavin, niacin, vitamin B6, pantothenic acid, iron, zinc, copper, manganese, and selenium.

Previously I had extremely painful period pain, which became unbearable as I became ill. I was barely able to walk some days, and often went into a type of shock where extreme nausea and shaking would take over my body. The pain became so unbearable throughout my worst years of stress and illness where I would often find myself hunched over my work desk, and once had to be carried out of my office and into a sick bay area. Since introducing cleansing superfoods to my lifestyle, my period pain has been mostly non-existent, and only noticeable when I have bad months of binging and stress and when I forget to drink wheatgrass. This learning I owe to Asian nutrition, specifically Paul Pitchford's *Healing with Wholefoods: Asian Traditions and Modern Nutrition*. This book started me on my journey to becoming a nutritional therapist. Thank you, Paul.

Although microalgae and wheatgrass are some of the most powerful superfoods on earth, there are many foods out there containing a higher amount of a particular micronutrient, which will specialize in your healing. Garlic, for example, has large amounts of allium, which are known to support blood and heart health by reducing the amount of cholesterol in the bloodstream. Ginger is known for its immune-boosting, digestive and anti-nausea properties. I always have a stash of these in my cupboard to incorporate into my cooking or to use as a remedy when I or someone else needs it.

Turmeric and cayenne pepper are also spices I always have in my food cupboard. Turmeric is a member of the curcumin family and is also a powerful antioxidant and anti-inflammatory, which helps to prevent heart disease, Alzheimer's and cancer. Cayenne chili pepper is a member of the capsaicin family, when consumed it speeds up the metabolism and can help the liver to heal. It is especially known for improving circulation. This has been well known in traditional Chinese and Ayurvedic medicine practices.

These are just a few examples of superfoods out there, and you will find many more with inquisition and need.

12
HEALTHIER TREAT FOODS

Living a healthy life isn't about cutting out everything you love and being boring. You want to live well and make the most of your life, while sustaining your health and well-being for ongoing happiness. Finding balance between the healthy and unhealthy is what's key and will be your challenge moving forward.

A good way to start is to find healthier alternatives for the things you love. If you love chowing down on a pizza and watching movies a few times a week, try switching it up to sourdough pizza and reducing your portion sizes. Make it a once-a-week occurrence, replacing a movie session with a swim or a trip to the gym. Adding more healthy alternatives to the mix will help balance everything out so you are healthier while still enjoying what you love.

One way I have found to keep my treats is to change them for healthier versions and reduce the portion sizes. I love chocolate and coffee, so now I only buy chocolate with at least sixty percent cocoa. This means I'm getting more nutrients (especially magnesium) and less unnatural fats and sugar. I even go for a high-quality brand containing more natural ingredients like cocoa butter and natural sugars. Having nuts in it also ensures it has more nutritional content and tastes great too!

I have switched to making my own coffee where I use fresh ground granules and mix it with goat milk and nut milk. This ensures I'm getting only natural and fresh ingredients and more nutrients from the milk. I have also reduced my consumption down to one coffee a day, and now I sometimes don't even want one.

Clear spirits are a better alternative to heavy sugar alcohols like beer and wine, although red wine (in small doses) has been shown to strengthen and cleanse the blood. Be careful some wines are laden with tannins, which are not good for the digestive system.

Almond butter is a great whole food to have stashed in your cupboard. You can mix it into stir-fries and use it to bake, as well as having it spread on rice cakes or sourdough with honey or healthy alternative chocolate spread. It is so versatile, and means you're getting a good dose of healthy unsaturated fats and B vitamins, which are good for your heart and brain health.

These are just a few ways I have switched up my treat foods for healthier alternatives, and it feels good to know I can always treat myself while still getting the nutrients I need. I share these with you, so you are able to benefit from a healthy lifestyle in a fun and enjoyable way.

13

POWERFUL TIPS FOR COMMENCING THE REVERSAL OF CHRONIC DISEASE SYMPTOMS RIGHT NOW

When you know there's something wrong, and you know you need to do something but are not entirely sure how, you can choose to focus on what you can control at the moment. Taking such action can produce immediate results and start the healing process for you straightaway. This is where your power lies.

Whether you're already learning about healing with nutrition or just thinking about it, start by simply stopping. Slow down and give yourself the time to allow learning, self-reflection and revision of any bad habits. It's not just about what you know but how you can use it to help yourself and possibly others.

When you know you need to do something about your health and life, you can immediately set the intention to receive all the support you need, so you can heal faster and more efficiently. No matter what that support looks like, it's important to first know and accept that you need it so you can begin to allow the healing to happen. What I'm saying is your mind is your first barrier, and thus tool, to real healing. All the knowledge in the world will not help you if you're not completely aligned to accepting where you are and what you need to heal. You will then be ready to see and accept the support you need to get your health where it needs to be.

For access to my online program, navigate to my portal *helenbarnshaw.podia.com*

To summarize:

- Slow down.
- Outline any bad habits.
- Get help to replace them with good habits.
- Allow support from a coach or resources to give you the most enjoyable and successful experience.
- Be completely honest with yourself and your expectations.
- Stay open-minded and keep learning.

14
TESTIMONIALS

One thing that has inspired me to write this guide is the experience I have had helping others. Some of these people were friends, some were family, and some were members of the public. All had different types and severity of illness, ranging from rheumatoid arthritis to Crohn's disease, to lower-level IBS symptoms. In each case, all that has been provided within this book is relevant to all of them, as a preventative measure and strategies for beginning reversal of symptoms and cause. They also each received a personally tailored diet and lifestyle strategy that gave them a solid footing to improve many areas of their lives, in addition to diet. The diet strategy is tailored to their body's specific nutrient requirements, metabolism, and disposition, with an optimum goal in mind. I call it the bible, as it provides them a range of information specifically tailored to them and to achieve optimal healing.

Hannah Pittaway, 2019

I saw Helen after being recommended by a friend. Helen is kind and supportive and I feel like she is always there if I need her or have any questions. After going through my deficiencies, I have a great strategy to follow with a list of foods that heal! The rest is up to me, but I know Helen is there with me all the way.

DEANNA BARNSHAW, 2018

I was diagnosed with aggressive rheumatoid disease three years ago—a chronic and progressive auto immune disorder which afforded me little relief from chronic pain. I decided to seek guidance and nutritional advice from Helen about six months ago. I am now pain free, my inflammation levels have decreased greatly, and I have been free from steroid treatment for two years. I feel that with Helen's advice I am gradually healing, she has lifted my spirits also. Supportive and calm in advising and gently guiding. I highly recommend!

PAUL PECCIOLI, 2019

Helen is passionate about her work and the people she is helping. Helen is committed to her clients and her work ethos in helping people have a better life and living. Helen is excellent at what she does, and I would recommend her highly in the knowledge that she is one of the best.

SPIRITUAL DEVELOPMENT GUIDANCE

15
INTENTION AND VISUALIZATION FOR SETTING OFF ON THE RIGHT PATH

I've gone through some of the most powerful habits and tools that have helped me and others succeed on our healing journeys. Everyone is different, and you will find many, if not all, chapters helpful on your journey.

When you develop the power of intention and start visualizing your higher self and what you want, you will naturally influence your healing direction. This is important if you are looking to achieve the fullest health and happiness for yourself. With true and powerful visualization and small steps, you will naturally go in the right direction. Every day, you will naturally attract and achieve specific steps towards your healing goals. You will quickly begin to see and feel the difference within yourself.

Setting an intention allows you to know exactly where you're going and get there faster; this creates fuller purpose. It helps you set the flow of direction more effortlessly, so you're not being swept away with life. It also helps you to reach your goals faster.

Meditation is the most powerful tool to help you when beginning on a road to intention setting. It helps to sit with your thoughts, and let them go, so you can learn to be more comfortable in trusting that there is a better way. As you begin to let go, you will start to feel your worries melt away; it is infinitely easier to visualize who you want to be and the things you want to achieve. This will allow you to begin to experience how you feel when you visualize your higher intentions. The more you allow yourself to feel the good things you want to feel, the more you are training your mind and body to accept being in that space now. It is as if you are already stepping into the visualization and your higher self. Feeling is the key here!

As Deepak Chopra tells us in *Creating Affluence*, "When we transcend, we know non-verbally, without the use of words. We obtain knowledge directly, without the distracting intervention of spoken language. This is the value of meditation, giving us the experience of pure being."

I HAVE NEVER TRIED VISUALIZATION BEFORE. HOW DO I BEGIN GETTING INTO THE MINDSET?

Start with gratitude for what you already have. When you can learn to see all the things you currently have, you then appreciate you are already blessed with opportunities. The more you train your mind to see things in this way, the more you naturally attract more of what you want. Again, it goes back to feeling, which is energy. This energy then naturally attracts more of the same energy. This is why it is so important to learn to focus your attention on the positive. Solidify these visualizations by writing them down, creating a mantra, sharing your intention with a close friend. Most importantly, feel how good you feel when you visualize your intentions. Be specific about what you want. Visualize how it looks and how you feel but don't focus on the details of how you'll get there. This is very important; let go and trust the universe to answer your call. When you try too hard to get what you want, what you actually end up doing is pushing your visualizations and higher purposes away, as you run towards activities based on your fears—of which you may not be aware.

Tools are a powerful way of strengthening your intention practice into action. Whether you use a digital or a paper diary, this is a strong way of noting thoughts, feelings, intentions, dreams and plans to help you to get there. By starting small and adding in a few tasks a day that align to your higher intentions, it supports you in the right direction, step by step. This will keep you on track and ensure you're always achieving the most specific activities on your journey.

I have created a Daily Habit Builder tool, which has helped some of my clients organize, plan, and achieve their highest healing daily and weekly goals. I will talk more about this in Chapter 18 and provide you with instructions on how to use it and its benefits to you. As mentioned earlier, meditation is a powerful tool. It has been one of the most useful tools in my kit for faster and sustainable healing, mainly because it reshapes your mind positively and supports faster habit building. I will share some techniques with you in the next chapter.

16
MEDITATION TO SUPPORT LASTING INFLUENCE ON YOUR MIND

Meditation is one of the most powerful tools out there at the moment. It has been used for centuries by Eastern cultures to practice peace of mind and gain spiritual healing. Meditation helps to calm the mind and develop our access to spiritual awareness—the soul intelligence. When your mind is calmer, your body is in better harmony. It is so highly recognized as a core well-being tool now that it is now used within schools to calm unruly behaviour in children.

Meditation will be one of your most powerful tools in your quest for healing. By relaxing your thinking mind and allowing yourself to let go of your expectations and how you think you should act, it opens up the way for your natural soul intelligence to influence you. Eckhart Tolle, in *The Power of Now*, explains that the thinking mind is the smaller self and the cause of learned bad habits and antiquated poor self-belief. The more you practice letting go through meditation, the more room there is for your brain to learn new and positive methods and the more your bodies and cells learn; this strengthens positive habit building. I believe it is the most powerful way to change habits. Changing habits cannot be attributed to knowledge alone, as without the will to want to make change, or the relevant tools to help your mind learn how to integrate this into your life, your efforts will be futile or even short-lived.

Your mind is the way you see and interact with the world. If you're going to attempt to change your habits, starting with your mind is the single most effective way to begin. There is no doubt meditation and therapy will help you here. There are many factors, which help build your mind to what it is today. Ancestry and evolution; family DNA and cells; birth environment; upbringing; food; exposure to toxins; and current environment. All of these factors have built your mind to what it is today. It is with the awareness of choice where you can begin to build better habits for a healthier and happier lifestyle. You are the one in control of your mind and when you begin to make small changes to your habits on a daily basis, you will start to see and feel your life experiences change. The more you do it, the bigger and longer lasting those changes are.

Meditation was first invented in India. It was seen in Indian wall art placed around 5000 to 3500 BCE. Evidence of the first written form was found in Vedas in 1500 BC. Meditation has seen growth through Japanese Buddhism and forms of yoga teaching which has extended to all over the world. In modern-day schools in Japan, meditation is used as a tool to support children's learning, development, and emotional health. The practice has now spread to Europe and the United States of America, as we see schools using it to support behavioural issues in children in place of detention and other antiquated disciplinary methods.

Meditation has been shown to reduce stress and help reprogram the brain in positive ways. It has been accepted as a positive therapy for anxiety and depression. Professional sports teams and military units are also using meditation to enhance performance. It has been shown to help sufferers of chronic pain and has been proven to reduce symptoms in cancer and HIV patients. MRI scans also show that after an eight-week course of meditation practice, the body's response to stress is reduced and the amygdala appears to shrink. This is the fear and emotion centre of the brain which usually results in the fight or flight response in people. You can find more information online through the National Centre for Biotechnology Information website. ncbi.nlm.nih.gov/pmc/articles/PMC5368208

I started using meditation for all of the reasons above on the commencement of my healing journey around four years ago. Back then I was suffering terrible symptoms of fibromyalgia with back, hip, leg and neck pain, chronic IBS, and hypoglycaemic attacks. The list goes on. The Headspace app—founded by Andy Puddicombe, who was taught as a Buddhist monk—led me to discover meditation groups and workshops. I now have a plethora of meditation techniques I use in the morning and sometimes during the day or at night if needed. As I have practiced meditation over the course of a few years now, it has become an effortless and very natural part of my life. Advanced meditation practice will support you in your everyday life and activities by helping you to achieve and stay in that space between thought and feeling; it helps you to let go. Just as it supports professional athletes within their performance, it will support you in everything you do. It is also for these reasons that I recommend it to those healing on my nutritional healing program. It is one of the most powerful tools to support you to be fully successful on your journey to full health and happiness.

Tips to Get You Started on Meditating at Home

Meditation apps: Download a mediation app like Headspace or Calm. These are designed to slowly introduce and guide you through the methods of meditation. With Headspace, you can start with a five-minute practice and build up to twenty minutes. You can choose what you want your meditation to focus on, so it focuses directly on a particular problem area to begin with, and it also has daily reminders and words of affirmation to keep you on track.

Meditation groups: Groups offer more advanced techniques of meditation, which help you to develop your practice into other areas of your life—such as walking and chanting meditation. As a development of Buddhist practice, it is a very rewarding way of meditating, as you share experiences with others and develop your positive energy on a group level, which is far more powerful than lone meditation. However, lone meditation offers its own strengths in being flexible and accessible to you whenever you need/want it.

Retreats: Retreats offer a development from group meditation, if this is what you're looking for. It is a more immersive experience. You will find this is a common method for teaching many highly advanced practices such as Vipassana meditation and yoga. It is a deeply mind-changing experience and quantum leap in spiritual evolvement. I have practiced up to three hours and am still working towards being able to do it for a whole day.

17
SELF-ACCEPTANCE AND SELF-COMPASSION: MAKING THE HEALING PROCESS EASIER

I hear this everywhere these days—self-compassion and self-love. It wasn't until I started to truly love myself and give myself a break and balance in everything I do, that I was able to really begin to heal on a deeper level. I began to feel the results of the love I was giving back to myself. In doing so, it has improved the care and support I share with others, as I teach them to heal and love themselves through nutrition, meditation and self-love.

In my own upbringing—and if you are an older generation—you were taught that failure is something you need to be afraid of and that it's not okay. This might have hindered you from being able to accept yourself as a fallible human being, who makes mistakes as a natural part of the human learning process. It is okay to do things that a human should do, because that is who you are. Schools now teach children that failure is part of the learning process. In doing so, we've been able to normalize failure as part of the natural learning process. This has made it easier for children to take steps towards being their true and best selves, without being afraid. Children are now able to achieve their dreams and desires sooner, shaping and influencing more positive and healthy adulthoods.

You and I are able to relearn these steps in order to understand the importance of self-love and acceptance in our healing process. Using meditation to support your mind and to let go of your thoughts and expectations of yourself, will help you to step away from any unhealthy habits which drive your daily actions. This is the age of retraining your mind to strengthen your healing journey and to sustain your health thereafter.

Talk to yourself about being okay with failure. Accept who you are. What do you love? What do you hate? What things are you afraid of? Write it all down. Look at it and know that what you feel when you look at these words, are feelings which you can change; in doing so, you are able to create new experiences of these things, in the age of relearning how to live better.

It's not until we allow ourselves to accept who we truly are, we can allow ourselves to let go and move through relearning and creating new experiences for ourselves.

Get support. Seek support from those around you, friends, family and others on a healing journey, as well as healers who are willing to support you on your journey. We are all here to learn from each other. No man is an island. When you can allow yourself to receive support, you can begin to see it and attract it everywhere. The universe is truly an amazing entity, and you are the universe. You and I are one, as corny as it sounds!

On my healing journey, I have sought support from everywhere—from therapists, other healers, trainers, friends, and even some members of my family. I realized while growing up I had been taught that seeking support from others was a sign of failure. When I was shown a better way—that it was okay and normal to get support from others—my healing made a quantum leap, bringing me fulfilment and happiness, which I was able to continue to share and teach to others.

I learned to accept myself wholly and that failures are all part of the journey we grow through as part of our learning and building process. I now no longer see failure as failure; I see it as a natural step in my process within anything I am achieving. That viewpoint allows me to let go and enjoy the process fully, learning from my mistakes and successes, informing me how best to move forward. It's a kind of natural directive—the universe showing me where to go. I fully accept this as a big part of the healing journey; when you are able to also see and accept this, you will begin to deeply connect with the process of self-love and healing.

HABIT-BUILDING TOOLS FOR HEALING

18
HOW PHYSICAL TOOLS MAKE IT EASIER TO BUILD POSITIVE HABITS

All the nutritional support and well-being methods in the world might not help you to fully heal if your mind is not healing and if you're not sure how to effectively implement the methods. Meditation deeply supports positive changes in your brain, materializing in better decision-making skills and reduced stress. Together with effective tools, you will experience much faster results as you learn the most successful ways to influence habit changes that will quantum leap your healing. The tips below are some of the best methods I have used for my own healing and to help others.

You want to start building this knowledge into bite size habits, which you can easily integrate into your daily life. Bringing everything you know into the real physical realm, you will quickly start to benefit from the rewards of symptom relief and deeper healing. Building positive habits is a way for you to quantum leap into the healing you desire, as it quickly bridges the gap between knowledge and the physical realm. It also offers more long-lasting learned behaviours, as you are able to quickly put into practice what does and doesn't work for you and are able to make changes more effectively to gain the faster results you're looking to gain.

Here are a few tools that I and many others have found particularly helpful:

Daily diary: To take the pressure from having to remember everything. It helps to know what to prioritize and get ahead on the areas you want to achieve first. Use it like a personal assistant.

Weekly shopping lists: To fully optimize the nutrients you need, and any herbal tinctures to reduce symptoms. Having a list has supported me to stay on track with what my body actually needs, rather than to veer off to buying what my mind thinks I need and giving in to temptations. In particular, I've always used a shopping app, adding what I need to my order on the go.

Apps to monitor macronutrients: I have clients who have discovered free apps to help them to monitor protein, fat and carbohydrate intake daily, more easily maximizing the nutrients from their personalized program. Macronutrients are the nutrients, which the body needs in larger amounts, to function. I have created a helpful tally chart which allows you to easily track these macro-nutrients in a daily diary format; it is included with a symptom monitoring guide.

Symptom tracker: A way of reminding yourself to monitor any reduction or rise in symptoms daily/weekly, for the purpose of seeing what's working or not working. From here you are able to more quickly identify any issues and make quick changes to rectify them, getting you back on track faster. The first couple of months being on a personalized nutritional therapy program is designed to support you and teach you about your body, build positive habits and helps keep you on track. I have created tools to help you to continue these

HABIT-BUILDING TOOLS FOR HEALING

positive habits outside of the program, so you have support even without me present.

Meal prepping: Meal prepping is when you cook up some of the ingredients in your fridge and make them into meals for the week ahead, then divide them out into portions. This makes the food more obtainable for you, as you've already got some meals and snacks prepped and ready to go! It is a good way of making it easier to obtain the nutrients you need and stay on track. It's too easy to binge when you don't have the foods you need. Meal prepping makes it easier for you to eat healthily and get what you need daily.

The Daily Habit Builder Tool: I created the Daily Habit Builder Tool to encompass all the very best features of the tools I had used and knew were helpful for others; It has helped to achieve the most optimal habits for nutrient intake and deep healing.

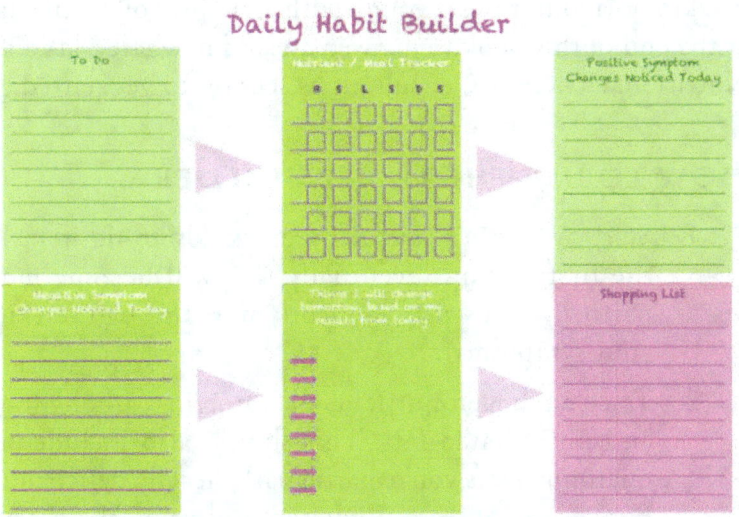

Fig 1.2, Daily Habit Builder Tool, download from helebarnshaw.podia.com

The tool is designed to be printed and used as it is. Stick it on your fridge or print out a few copies and staple together as a make-shift diary or copy the singular elements of the tool that you feel you need, into your diary. This will support the format of your daily routine to keep you deeply focused and on track. Think of it as your personal PA to support you.

Use the tool daily or weekly to keep you on track with specific guidance and actions. I found it helpful to use the elements in my diary on a weekly basis—dedicating thirty minutes of my time once a week. This then gave me specific actions to go away with for the next week, which kept me on the right path towards my health goals. This will make life easier for you, and people will wonder how you're achieving your healing with such ease.

If using the tool to heal more chronic illness and stress, it is much more effective alongside a tailored nutritional therapy program. Without this, you won't have the deeper knowledge of what you're deficient in and why, and what you specifically need to do about it to set your health straight. Follow the link at the end of this book to my website and navigate to the 1-1 Nutritional Therapy Consultations section to get started.

How to use the Habit Builder

1. Start by writing your daily or weekly to-do items in the first section (eventually this will become more narrowly focused as you work more through tracking your symptoms).

2. Track any macronutrients like protein, carbohydrate, and unsaturated fats. This should also include any micronutrients you're particularly heavily deficient in. For chronic disease, I advise monitoring these daily. The more you do it, the more natural it will become to you, and eventually you won't need the tool.

HABIT-BUILDING TOOLS FOR HEALING

3. Give yourself some time to work through any positive changes you've noticed today/this week. Example: it could be that you're noticing more energy—this might be due to you eating more complex carbs and sleeping better. Or it may be that you've replaced refined sugar and carbonated drinks with natural sugars, which means your digestion is feeling lighter and your skin may be clearer.

4. Do the same for any negative symptom changes you notice daily or weekly. What feelings haven't subsided? Although some symptoms may take a while to lessen, the more you do to reduce them, the faster you'll see positive changes. Sometimes doing two or three things might tackle a whole heap of symptoms at once. If you find these symptoms stubborn, due to more chronic illness, there are natural remedies, which will help you to reduce the negative symptoms, while you're learning better behaviours and habits and healing yourself on a cellular level. I have supplied an introduction to some of the best herbs and tinctures to get you started. You'll find books just on this category alone.

5. In this section, note things you want to change and some direct actions you will do to get this rolling. For example, you may want to speed up your brain fog reduction. You may want to do this through reducing stress at work, getting more sleep, eating more plant-based foods with high amounts of chlorophyll to detox the gut (see the gut-mind connection chapter for more info). Or you might want to start eating more vitamin B foods to help increase Serotonin and neurological cell production and support.

6. Buy any wholefoods and herbs that you want to add to your nutritional profile and daily diet. It might be

that you already have these, and you want to top up before you run out.

Either way, this tool has been designed from the best tips and strategies to help you (as it has helped others and myself) to stay focused and on track with your health goals. You will begin to experience reduced symptoms, reverse illness, and prevent onset of more chronic disease.

You can find this Habit Builder Tool at *helenbarnshaw.podia.com* along with other downloads and video courses to fast track your healing. All the information in the world can't help us until we know how to turn it into practical and real healing.

ABOUT THE AUTHOR

Around 2016 I became ill with chronic body pain in the form of Fibromyalgia, Irritable Bowel Syndrome (IBS), stomach ulcers, and hyperglycaemic attacks. This was an accumulation of minor symptoms I had already been experiencing over a period of years and—as I would soon learn—was connected to my environment, upbringing, and family history. Although I was using different forms of pharmaceutical medication and attending traditional osteopathic sessions for my spinal pain, I was still stuck in a never-ending spiral of, what seemed to be, no way out.

I've always been a practical, hands-on, get-things-done sort of a person due to my regimented upbringing. Although I was trying to teach myself to slow down and accept as much help as I could to heal, I realized there was more to fuller, longer-term healing than simply popping a pill or sitting in an osteopath's chair. I decided to seek some deeper, inner healing through meditation, psychological therapy, and naturopathic nutrition. I started tackling my negative self-image through therapy and rebirthing my mind, but I also knew I needed to understand how to reverse some of the damage I'd already done to my body and to speed up its healing. I wanted to start experiencing the benefits of deeper healing sooner rather than later, so I could make the most of my new-found self-compassion and self-love in creating the best life for myself. The more I learned and tested on myself, the more I experienced progressive healing, which enlivened my happiness and empowered my soul. I realized I had to start questioning traditional methods as a way of healing fully. I suspected traditional methods had kept others and me in a place of stubborn pain and anxiety. Although traditional medicine does have a place in an emergency, I believe it does not have to be a long-term solution. When we learn to see and trust naturopathic nutrition as a better way of healing, we begin to jump beyond our current limits of expectation and happiness, and we experience unprecedented levels of suspended health, wealth, power, and happiness.

As I went deeper into my meditation practice, I discovered how to love others and myself more powerfully. This led me to naturopathic nutrition as a more natural and long-term solution for pain relief and fuller healing. I started by reading about Asian traditions and whole foods, which taught me the best of the Asian methods of naturopathy. They have been used for decades and have started to influence modern naturopathy. As I read, I tested the methods on myself—first successfully reducing my symptoms of IBS and then reducing all other chronic symptoms. The more I saw and felt it working, the more I believed in it as a better and lasting way of healing to fuller happiness. I wanted to learn more. From there I received a western naturopathic nutrition diploma. After successful completion of the exam and real practice on others, I felt confident enough to share with and help others who really needed it. I wanted to empower others to see a better, faster, and long-lasting way of physical and emotional healing for fuller well-being.

I started to help those around me who I could see wanted the support. My mother, who has rheumatoid arthritis, friends in a local fibromyalgia group, colleagues at work, friends of friends and other new clients who were recommended to my

ABOUT THE AUTHOR

services. I am especially interested in helping people integrate functional healing—healing with whole foods—in an easy and hassle-free way, allowing them to make small, manageable changes one step at a time. These small changes eventually become lasting habits, resulting in faster symptom reduction and healing on a cellular level.

I found it helpful to use a balance of what is already available to us in the well-being market and homemade recipes. I share with others time-saving tips that use functional foods and tinctures—herb and spice medicine mixtures—to reduce symptoms fast and heal long term. I believe genuine healing is about making solutions real and accessible. Healing is not an unreachable thing for only people with money and time to spare. It is for everyone, and it is here for us now. You'll need to see it, want to achieve it, and accept yourself on the journey. Healing is not an overnight fix. It's a state of mind and a belief system that takes us beyond traditional archetypal methods. There is such a wealth of knowledge out there now, you will find everything you're looking for if you're ready to accept and embark on the journey to fuller healing. You are starting right here with this accessible, coaching book.

APPENDICES

BIBLIOGRAPHY

Chapter 2
IICT Nutritional Therapy Practitioner Diploma. The Health Sciences Academy. US. 2018.

Nicolle, Lorraine. Beirne, Ann Woodriff. *Biochemical Imbalances in Disease: A Practitioner's Handbook.* London: Singing Dragon, 2010.

Chapter 3
Nicolle, Lorraine. Beirne, Woodriff. *Biochemical Imbalances in Disease: A Practitioner's Handbook.* London: Singing Dragon, 2010.

Narby, Jeremy. *Intelligence in Nature.* New York: Penguin Group, 2005.

Chapter 7
Narby, Jeremy. *Intelligence in Nature.* New York: Penguin Group, 2005.

Chapter 11
Pitchford, Paul. *Healing with Wholefoods: Asian Traditions and Modern Nutrition.* US: North Atlantic Books, 2002.

Chapter 15
Barnshaw, Helen. *Daily Habit Builder Tool.* 2019.
Chopra, Deepak. *Creating Affluence.* San Rafael, CA: New World Library, 1993.

Chapter 16
Tolle, Eckhart. *Practising the Power of Now: Meditations, Exercises and Core Teachings from The Power of Now.* UK: Yellow Kite, 2016.

Hilton L, Hempel S, Ewing BA, et al. "Mindfulness Meditation for Chronic Pain: Systematic Review and Meta-analysis." *Annals of behavioral medicine: a publication of the Society of Behavioral Medicine* vol. 51,2 (2017): 199-213. doi:10.1007/s12160-016-9844-2. Accessed via *NCBI* website. ncbi.nlm.nih.gov/pmc/articles/PMC5368208.

ADDITIONAL TOOLS AND RESOURCES

You can find additional downloads and videos to guide and support you throughout your whole healing journey, on my portal *helenbarnshaw.podia.com*

It's easy to access and get started.

In the portal you will find useful self-test sheets, a habit-builder tool, and extensive video courses to support you at every step of your healing. You can use the downloadable sheets to support you with the practical chapters in this book, and you can use the course videos to continue and supplement your learning journey even further. This is for people ready for Healing Guru status!

Remember, this book is a solid base to get started on your healing journey and using the resources will help you to make it a reality. All the information in the world won't help us until we actually turn it into practice. These additional tools will help you to easily get started as soon as possible and will continue to support and guide you throughout the rest of your healing journey.

ONLINE PROGRAM

If you're experiencing some sort of digestive issue (IBS, IBD, Chrohn's Disease etc), bodily infections, feeling fatigued all the time, regular colds & flu, slow wound healing, or you suffer from high stress levels, here is your next best step to begin reversing some of your symptoms and strengthening your body. These provide you with step-by-step guidance to achieve your best health. They are designed to powerfully kick-start your healing journey, quantum leaping you to healing on a cellular level, reducing stress, reducing pain, improving sleep, losing weight, or just improving your core functional health to strengthen your defences against harmful microbes and virus'.

Follow me on social media for more information and daily tips:

instagram.com/hbarnshawnutritionalhealing

facebook.com/HBarnshawNutritionalHealing

talkhealthpartnership.com/blog/author/helen-barnshaw

ENDORSEMENTS

A must-have pocket coach for anyone on a healing journey. I like the simplicity of information presented in this book. I relate to it well as a Chinese woman, especially around Yin and Yang food and use of herbal for healing.

—Yuliana Hartanto
Energy Healer and Transformational Coach
at Life Path Alchemist

Good read, with easy techniques to boost you on your healing journey. Everyone is busy these days, but don't forget to pause for thought. Helen guides you through some simple but devastatingly effective steps to integrate functional healing into your normal routine, helping you to build good habits that stick.

—Neil Golding
Marine Scientist

www.ingramcontent.com/pod-product-compliance
Lightning Source LLC
LaVergne TN
LVHW021944060526
838200LV00042B/1919